MW00572927

Healthy
Expectations

Healthy
Expectations

Pamela Smith, R.D.

Healthy Expectations—
a Daily Journal for Expectant Mothers
by Pamela Smith

Published by Creation House
Strang Communications Company
600 Rinehart Road
Lake Mary, Florida 32746
Web site: http://www.creationhouse.com

Unless otherwise noted, all Scripture quotations are from the Holy Bible, New International Version. Copyright © 1973, 1978, 1984, International Bible Society. Used by permission.

Scripture quotations marked KJV are from the King James Version of the Bible.

Scripture quotations marked NAS are from the New American Standard Bible. Copyright © 1960, 1962, 1963, 1968, 1971, 1972, 1973, 1975, 1977 by the Lockman Foundation. Used by permission.

Scripture quotations marked TLB are from The Living Bible. Copyright © 1971. Used by permission of Tyndale House Publishers Inc., Wheaton, IL 60189. All rights reserved.

Smith, Pamela M.
    Health expectations journal: preparing a healthy body for a
healthy baby/ Pamela Smith.
        p.   cm.
    ISBN 0-88419-527-9 (hardback)
    1. Pregnancy. 2. Pregnancy—Nutritional aspects. 3. Pregnancy—
Religous aspects. I. Title.
RG525.S625   1998
618.2'4—dc21
                                                                98-2913
                                                                CIP

Printed in the United States of America
89012345 / BVG / 87654321

To my two amazing daughters
Danielle and Nicole:
You fill my heart with joy and wonder and
bless my life with your tender love.
Life with you has exceeded
my greatest expectations.
I thank God for the precious gift of you,
and for allowing me to be your mother.

Dear Mom-to-be,

New life has been created inside you, and you have been given a special privilege—the joy of nurturing your baby within until birth! The months of pregnancy are some of the most incredible months of a woman's life. From the moment the possibility of being pregnant becomes an awesome reality, you are thrust into months of wonder and anticipation.

Take time every day to reflect on your pregnancy. Journal your feelings and thoughts—it's a wonderful time for you to think about and put into words what you are experiencing. It is also a wonderful way to make this more than a pregnancy—a wonderful, personal story about the birthing of your baby—and the birthing of you as a mother.

If you are like me, you may feel hesitant about journaling. No time, no privacy, nothing to write about. Your time of pregnancy is a perfect time to lay those protests aside...you have a very focused subject to write about, a bursting dam of feelings to be felt, and an incredible opportunity to record a miracle. That's why I wanted to offer you this very special chance to record your pregnancy experience in this Healthy Expectations Journal—perhaps to be able to share with your child someday. You may also want to get a copy of my book, *Healthy Expectations*—the companion to this journal.

As you begin to write, your self-consciousness will fade, enabling you to write more easily the feelings, thoughts, and fears that flood your inner soul and spirit. You can write about your joys, regrets, hopes, inadequacies, exciting happenings, moans and groans, happy thoughts, or what the baby did that day.

Find a few quiet moments—the last few before slipping into sleep or the first few moments after awakening. Or, close the door, unplug the phone, and sit quietly for a few uninterrupted moments to reflect on the struggles and joys of each day through journaling. Then close your eyes, take a deep breath, and put your hands over your womb. Send heart messages of love to your baby—rejoicing in the miracle of God.

The beauty of the written word is that it can be held close to the heart and read over and over again.
— FLORENCE LITTAUER

7

Father, I thank You for my unborn child. I treasure this child as a gift from You.
My child was created in Your image, perfectly healthy and complete.
You have known my child since conception and know the path my child will take in life.
I ask Your blessing, and stand in faith, believing Your plan for my child.

A HEALTHY EXPECTATION
+ + + + + + +

The months of pregnancy are some of the most incredible months of a woman's life.
Your time of pregnancy is not only the knitting together of the baby, it is a preparation
for your glorious new life, for the new emotional and spiritual you—a time to build
healthy expectations for your body, heart, and soul.

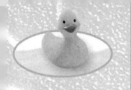

He will love you and bless you and increase your numbers. He will bless the fruit of your womb.

—DEUTERONOMY 7:13

A HEALTHY EXPECTATION

◆ ◆ ◆ ◆ ◆ ◆ ◆

New life has been created inside you, and you have been given a special privilege—the joy of nurturing your baby within until birth! Eating well is a way to express your love for your baby right from the very start. Good nutrition is the gift that only you can give your baby, but that gift goes on—and keeps on giving!

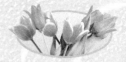

A baby is God's opinion that life should go on . . .

—CARL SANDBURG

_____
_____
_____
_____
_____
_____
_____
_____
_____
_____
_____
_____
_____
_____
_____
_____
_____
_____
_____
_____
_____

A HEALTHY EXPECTATION
+ + + + + + +

The First Day: Today a single-cell organism was formed in the image of God through the union of you and Dad-to-be. Over the coming months, your son or daughter will develop from this barely visible cell, called a *zygote*. This beginning is called *conception*. Over the next nine to ten days, your baby will travel through the uterus (home for the next eight-and-a-half-months), and will begin to grow rapidly, doubling in size every twenty-four hours.

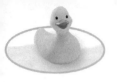

Blessed is he whose help is the God of Jacob, whose hope is in the Lord his God, the Maker of heaven and earth, the sea, and everything in them— the Lord who remains faithful forever.

—PSALM 146:5–6

_____

_____

_____

_____

_____

_____

_____

_____

_____

_____

_____

_____

_____

_____

_____

_____

_____

_____

_____

A HEALTHY EXPECTATION

✦ ✦ ✦ ✦ ✦ ✦ ✦

Yes, it takes a conscious effort to provide your baby with the very best. No maternal instinct draws you to a good diet and keeps you from what is harmful, but the reward of a healthy baby and child is far worth the effort!

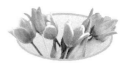

It is futile to wish
for a long life, and
then to give so little
care to living well!

—THOMAS A' KEMPIS

A HEALTHY
EXPECTATION

✦ ✦ ✦ ✦ ✦ ✦ ✦

Good health habits
have never been
more important
than they are right
now. If you are the
type of person who
already eats well-
balanced meals,
exercises
moderately, gets
sufficient rest, and
does not drink
alcohol or take
drugs, stay the
course. If you need
an excuse to finally
take better care of
yourself, let your
baby be that
excuse. Any
positive changes at
any time during
your pregnancy
benefit both you
and baby.

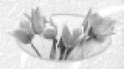

Your child has many hidden treasures that, once uncovered, polished, and held up to the light of encouragement, will lead him to success.

—ERIC BUEHRER

_____

_____

_____

_____

_____

_____

_____

_____

_____

_____

_____

_____

_____

_____

_____

_____

_____

_____

_____

A HEALTHY EXPECTATION

✦ ✦ ✦ ✦ ✦ ✦ ✦

Think of pregnancy as a twelve month experience—a minimum of three months to
prepare a healthy body for a healthy baby—and nine months to build a strong baby
with food and love. It is also just a beginning—because not only is a baby being
brought into the world, so is a mother.

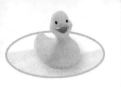

You [and your child]
are very special and
unique. No one on
earth has your
fingerprints. Therefore,
that makes you
"thumbbody."

—AL BRICE

_____

_____

_____

_____

_____

_____

_____

_____

_____

_____

_____

_____

_____

_____

_____

_____

_____

_____

_____

_____

A HEALTHY
EXPECTATION
✦ ✦ ✦ ✦ ✦ ✦ ✦
We now have
exciting evidence
showing that your
healthy eating
before, and during,
pregnancy not only
impacts the very
growth and
development of
your little one, but
prevents birth
defects and impacts
your baby's
immunity system
and chemical
balance, even his
intelligence,
throughout his
growing years.

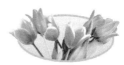

Yet, O Lord, you are our Father. We are the clay, you are the potter;
we are all the work of your hand.

—ISAIAH 64:8

Lord, I trust that You are molding this baby's physical body perfectly according to Your divine plan. Mold his mind and spirit also as he is formed. Mold me into the mother You have created me to be.

A HEALTHY EXPECTATION

✦ ✦ ✦ ✦ ✦ ✦ ✦

Every human needs protein, carbohydrates, vitamins, minerals, water, and even fat (in limited amounts); pregnancy only intensifies the need. In order to support the tremendous amount of growth and development that takes place during these special nine months, you will need a diet sufficient in calories and rich in nutrients.

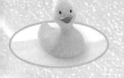

*Blessed art thou
among women, and
blessed is the fruit of
thy womb.*

—LUKE 1:42, KJV

Thank You, Father,
for the gift of this
incredible life
within me—thank
You for blessing
me with such
miraculous fruit.

_____

_____

_____

_____

_____

_____

_____

_____

_____

_____

_____

_____

_____

_____

_____

_____

_____

_____

_____

_____

_____

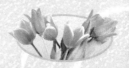

I praise you because I am fearfully and wonderfully made;
your works are wonderful, I know that full well.

—PSALM 139:14

A HEALTHY EXPECTATION

+ + + + + + +

Selecting a practitioner may be a most difficult task. You need to weigh many considerations as you choose the person who will direct the medical course of your pregnancy and attend the birth of your baby. Most importantly, do you feel a connection and rapport with this very important person; do you feel a freedom to share what's important to you?

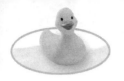

God, You who crafted the universe, have also marvelously designed my body to carry and birth my baby. I thank You, God, You who made the heavens and the earth and everything in them, will provide for the perfect growth and development of my baby. Amen.

A touch of
queasiness may be
your first clue that
you are pregnant.
The exact cause of
morning sickness is
simply unknown.
What is known is
that it is not
restricted to the
morning. It is also
known that fatigue,
stress, and a diet
low in vitamins,
minerals, and
carbohydrates can
make early-
pregnancy nausea
even more severe.
Also known:
An even, frequent
intake of low-fat
proteins balanced
with carbohydrates
throughout the day
will help to keep
your blood sugars
stable and prevent
the quease before it
hits!

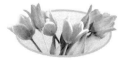

He has the film of my whole life in view, not just the snapshot of my present situation.

—W. TROBLISCH

A HEALTHY EXPECTATION
* * * * * * *

Gaining weight at a steady rate, and keeping the gain within the recommended
levels (twenty-five to thirty-five pounds), can greatly improve your odds of
escaping or minimizing such misery factors as hemorrhoids, varicose veins,
stretch marks, backaches, fatigue, heartburn, and shortness of breath.

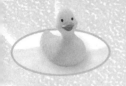

*The Lord . . .
will strengthen
your frame.*

—ISAIAH 58:11

Ask God for His
strength as this
baby is growing
within and putting
much pressure
upon every part
of your body.
Believe Him to
guide you into
caring for your
body and keeping
it strong.

A HEALTHY
EXPECTATION
✦ ✦ ✦ ✦ ✦ ✦ ✦
Getting enough of
the right kind of
exercise can help
improve your
overall well-being.
Exercise is
important at any
time, but especially
in repeat
pregnancies;
abdominal muscles
tend to be laxer,
making you more
susceptible to lots
of aches and pains.

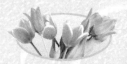

I will instruct you in the way you should go; I counsel you and watch over you.

—Psalm 32:8

_____

_____

_____

_____

_____

_____

_____

_____

_____

_____

_____

_____

_____

_____

_____

_____

A HEALTHY EXPECTATION
✦ ✦ ✦ ✦ ✦ ✦ ✦

You will need approximately three hundred extra calories per day while you are
pregnant. You may need a little less in the first trimester, and a little more in the last.
But your vitamin and mineral needs jump as much as 25 to 100 percent. That is why
what you eat is as vital as _how much_ you eat.

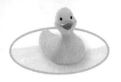

Children ... they string our joys, like jewels bright, upon the thread of years.

—EDWARD A. GUEST

_____

_____

_____

_____

_____

_____

_____

_____

_____

_____

_____

_____

_____

_____

_____

_____

_____

_____

_____

_____

_____

_____

_____

_____

_____

A HEALTHY
EXPECTATION
+ + + + + + +
Your best bet is
NOT to count
calories, but to
simply focus on
eating nutritious
foods at the right
times, in the right
balance. Your
appetite will come
into balance as
well, when you
begin to meet the
demands of the
pregnancy with the
proper foods.

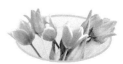

37

Just as there comes a warm sunbeam into every cottage window, so comes a love—born of God's care for every separate need.

—NATHANIAL HAWTHORNE

A HEALTHY EXPECTATION
+ + + + + + +

Although it may not seem like new news, breakfast still is the most important meal of your day—don't leave home without it! If you want to start your day with a boundless energy level, your metabolism in high gear, and proteins actively building you and your baby's new cells, then never skip breakfast!

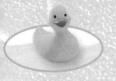

It is of the Lord's mercies that we are not consumed, because his compassions fail not. They are new every morning.

—LAMENTATIONS 3:22, KJV

God, thank You that each day begins anew— with fresh health and strength from You.

_____

_____

_____

_____

_____

_____

_____

_____

_____

_____

_____

_____

_____

_____

_____

_____

_____

_____

_____

A HEALTHY EXPECTATION

✦ ✦ ✦ ✦ ✦ ✦ ✦

Eat breakfast soon after you get up (within the first half-hour of arising). Go light and easy if time is a push; try some eat-and-go meals like fresh fruit and skim-milk shakes, cheese melted on whole wheat toast, and fruit, or freshly fruited yogurt with a homemade muffin or cereal.

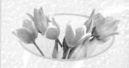

List of parental requirements: Affection without sentiment, authority without cruelty, discipline without aggression, humor without ridicule, sacrifice without obligation, companionship without possessiveness.

—WILLIAM E. BLATZ

_____

_____

_____

_____

_____

_____

_____

_____

_____

_____

_____

_____

_____

_____

_____

_____

_____

_____

_____

_____

_____

_____

_____

_____

_____

_____

_____

_____

_____

_____

_____

_____

_____

_____

_____

_____

A HEALTHY EXPECTATION
✦ ✦ ✦ ✦ ✦ ✦ ✦

Try to eat consistently and evenly each day, including three meals with at least two
healthy snacks. Ideally, you should eat 25 percent of your calories at breakfast,
25 percent at lunch, 25 percent at dinner, and the other 25 percent in healthy snacks.

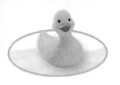

When I approach a
child, he inspires in
me two sentiments:
tenderness for what
he is, and respect for
what he may become.

—LOUIS PASTEUR

_____

_____

_____

_____

_____

_____

_____

_____

_____

_____

_____

_____

_____

_____

_____

_____

_____

_____

_____

_____

The Seventh week:
The chest and
abdomen are
completely formed.
The mouth opens;
there are tiny shell-
like external ears.
All of the backbone
is laid down, and
the spinal canal is
closed over. Arms
and legs are
beginning to be
visible. The baby is
now one-half-inch
long and weighs
one-thousandth of
an ounce.

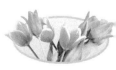

He gives strength to the weary and increases the power of the weak . . .
those who hope in the Lord will renew their strength.

—ISAIAH 40:29, 31

A HEALTHY EXPECTATION
+ + + + + + +

Keep power snacks available wherever you are—in your car, your desk drawer, your briefcase, a purse, or a diaper bag! They can be as simple as fresh fruit or a box of raisins with low-fat cheese or yogurt, a half sandwich, or even a trail mixture of dry roasted peanuts, sunflower seeds, and dried fruit.

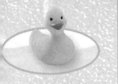

The best inheritance
a parent can give
her children is a few
minutes of her time
each day.

—O. A. BATTISTA

_____

_____

_____

_____

_____

_____

_____

_____

_____

_____

_____

_____

_____

_____

_____

_____

_____

_____

_____

_____

_____

A HEALTHY EXPECTATION

* * * * * * *

A healthy snack provides you with needed nutrition and will keep your blood-sugar level from dropping too low, leaving you sleepy and craving sweets. It will keep your metabolism burning high, with your and your baby's needs satisfied, and still not load you down with unwanted, unneeded fat, salt, sugar, and calories.

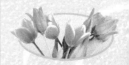

... all the time we wondered and wondered—who is this person
coming/growing/turning/floating/swimming deep, deep inside.

—CRESCENT DRAGONWAGON

A HEALTHY EXPECTATION

✦ ✦ ✦ ✦ ✦ ✦ ✦

Balance is vital to utilizing nutrients optimally. And balance is more than just a pretty plate—it's getting the right foods at the right time—always including carbohydrates and proteins at every meal and snack.

51

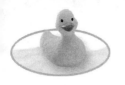

It is possible to give without loving, but it is impossible to love without giving.

—R. BRAUNSTEIN

_____

_____

_____

_____

_____

_____

_____

_____

_____

_____

_____

_____

_____

_____

_____

_____

_____

_____

_____

_____

_____

A HEALTHY EXPECTATION

✦ ✦ ✦ ✦ ✦ ✦ ✦

Carbohydrate-containing foods, and the nutrients they contain, are essential to your baby's growth and development. Whole grain-carbohydrates are particularly valuable because they have not had the outer layers of grain removed—they contain many more vitamins, minerals, and fiber than the refined, white products.

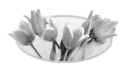

You knit me together in my mother's womb.

—PSALM 139:13

Thank You, Lord, for this baby being knit together perfectly,
according to Your perfect design. Thank You that I can rejoice that this baby
is the result of Your engineering, not by chance, not by accident.

A HEALTHY EXPECTATION

Folic acid is now known to be crucial for preventing neural tube birth defects such as spina bifida. It is so important that most physicians recommend that their patients supplement their diets with four hundred micrograms of folic acid for the three month's before conception and also throughout pregnancy. In addition, meet your need for this valuable nutrient with two servings of fresh, dark green, leafy veggies each day. Remember—if they're loaded with color, they're loaded with nutrition.

Children and
chickens would ever
be eating.

—THOMAS TUSSER

_____

_____

_____

_____

_____

_____

_____

_____

_____

_____

_____

_____

_____

_____

_____

_____

_____

_____

_____

Your need for
protein increases
greatly during
pregnancy. It is the
"new you," and it
becomes a building
block for you and
your baby's new
cells. The brain cell
development of
your baby depends
on your protein
intake—as does
the growth of the
uterus and
placenta.

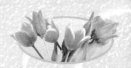

The future destiny of the child is always the work of the mother.

—NAPOLEON

Lord, as I am being prepared to be birthed as a mother, You know the pressures I feel, You know the concerns and fears I have. I cast these cares upon You, and pray for Your guidance and wisdom.

_____

_____

_____

_____

_____

_____

_____

_____

_____

_____

_____

_____

_____

_____

_____

_____

_____

_____

_____

_____

_____

_____

_____
_____
_____
_____
_____
_____
_____
_____
_____
_____
_____
_____
_____
_____
_____
_____
_____
_____
_____
_____
_____
_____

A HEALTHY EXPECTATION
+ + + + + + +

Protein boosts your metabolism, building body muscles and nerve tissue, as well as
providing for growth of the placenta and uterus. It serves to keep body fluids in
balance (excessive swelling and fluid retention is often caused by inadequate protein)
and makes beautiful hair, skin, and nails for your baby and you!

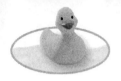

God loves us the way
we are, but He loves
us too much to leave
us that way.

—LEIGHTON FORD

A HEALTHY EXPECTATION

+ + + + + + +

A particularly wise choice for low-fat proteins while pregnant is fish—an excellent source of omega-3 fatty acids. These good-for-you oils have been shown to protect the heart, ease rheumatoid arthritis pain—and even improve infants' IQs (good news: Omega-3s are also found in breast milk). Omega-3s may also reduce the chances of premature birth and low birth weight.

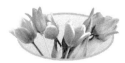

And we know that in all things God works for the good of those who love him, who have been called according to his purpose.

—ROMANS 8:28

_____

_____

_____

_____

_____

_____

_____

_____

_____

_____

_____

_____

_____

_____

_____

_____

_____

_____

_____

_____

_____

_____

_____

_____

A HEALTHY EXPECTATION

* * * * * * *

Pregnancy can give a sense of freedom to eat fat-laden foods with abandon—feeling
you're already fat, so what matter? Remember that there is a big difference between
being fat and being pregnant! The healthy foods you eat are making you and your baby
healthy; the excess fat you eat only breeds more work for you after delivery.

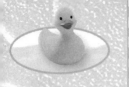

Each child is
an adventure into
a better life,
an opportunity
to change the
old pattern and
make it new.

—HUBERT H. HUMPHREY

The Twelfth week:
At this time, your
precious bundle of
joy is now three
inches long and
weighs one whole
ounce. Arms, legs,
hands, feet, fingers,
and toes are fully
formed. Nails
appear. The brain,
spinal cord, and
muscles connect,
and the baby can
kick those tiny legs
even though the
movement cannot
be felt yet. That
sweet thing can
make a fist, open
its mouth, and
squint those eyes.

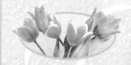

A human being is happiest and most successful when dedicated to a cause outside his own individual, selfish satisfaction.

—BENJAMIN SPOCK

A HEALTHY EXPECTATION
+ + + + + + +

Should you "just say no" to that diet soda? How about that morning cup of coffee with all of its caffeine? And what should you sweeten that ice tea with? I consider the best posture to be, "When in doubt, leave it out!" After all, it's only nine months—but nine months that will impact your baby's life, and yours—forever.

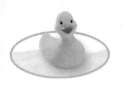

*Good health to you
and your household!
And good health to
all that is yours!*

—1 SAMUEL 25:6

Lord, thank You for
Your blessings of
good health and
strength for me and
my growing child
within.

_____

_____

_____

_____

_____

_____

_____

_____

/

_____

_____

_____

_____

_____

_____

_____

_____

_____

_____

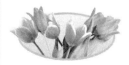

Faith is the inborn capacity to see God behind everything.

—OSWALD CHAMBERS

A HEALTHY EXPECTATION

♦ ♦ ♦ ♦ ♦ ♦ ♦

Establishing a healthy relationship with food now, while you're pregnant, provides
the framework for modeling a healthy attitude to your growing child about food.
Remember that your attitudes about eating are a significant contribution to your
little one's health.

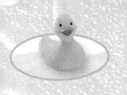

The desire to fulfill
the purpose for which
we were created is a
gift from God.

—A. W. TOZER

_____

_____

_____

_____

_____

_____

_____

_____

_____

_____

_____

_____

_____

_____

_____

_____

_____

_____

_____

_____

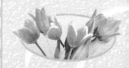

When one door closes, another opens, but we often look so long and so regretfully upon the closed door that we do not see the one that has opened for us.

—ALEXANDER GRAHAM BELL

_____

_____

_____

_____

_____

_____

_____

_____

_____

_____

_____

_____

_____

_____

_____

_____

A HEALTHY EXPECTATION
+ + + + + + +
Calcium is necessary to keep your own bones and teeth strong, and is needed for the
skeletal development in your baby. Every hour of the day throughout your pregnancy,
your baby draws calcium from your body's supply. Eating enough high calcium foods is
particularly crucial in the last three months of pregnancy when the baby's bone
formation is taking place at an accelerated rate.

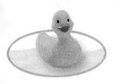

All that I am, or
hope to be, I owe to
my angel mother.

—ABRAHAM LINCOLN

_____

_____

_____

_____

_____

_____

_____

_____

_____

_____

_____

_____

_____

_____

_____

_____

_____

_____

_____

_____

_____

_____

A HEALTHY
EXPECTATION
+ + + + + + +
Along with your
needs for protein,
zinc, and calcium
increasing, you
must be careful to
eat enough foods
high in iron.
Because so much
iron is needed
during pregnancy a
supplement is
almost always
prescribed by your
physician as a form
of insurance.
Include food
sources highest in
iron, most notably:
dried apricots,
prunes, prune juice,
dried beans, whole
grains, well-cooked
oysters and clams,
and lean red meats
and poultry.

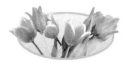

One reason for doing the right things today . . . is tomorrow!

—ANONYMOUS

A HEALTHY EXPECTATION
+ + + + + + +
Are you following the Eat Well, Live Well Prescription? Are you eating the right foods,
at the right time, in the right balance, with lots of brightly colored fruits and
vegetables? Start your day with breakfast, and eat evenly distributed "minimeals"
throughout your day.

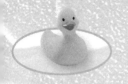

Heavenly Father,
Energize me and
help me to carve
out the time for
exercise and self-
care—keeping my
eyes focused on
strengthening my
physical body.

_____

_____

_____

_____

_____

_____

_____

_____

_____

_____

_____

_____

_____

_____

_____

_____

_____

_____

_____

_____

_____

_____

_____

A HEALTHY EXPECTATION
✦ ✦ ✦ ✦ ✦ ✦ ✦
Are you exercising? Instead of depleting your resources, exercise increases your energy. Just as it makes your metabolism and heart work better, exercise helps the brain function more efficiently. It also has a powerful anti-depressant effect to chase the blues away by boosting endorphins.

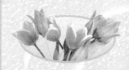

An ounce of prevention is worth a pound of cure.

—ANONYMOUS

A HEALTHY EXPECTATION
+ + + + + + +

My answer to the weight-gain question is a simple one: The healthiest babies are born
to women who allow themselves a natural weight gain during pregnancy. No matter
what your weight was before you conceived, you must have additional nutrient intake
to support an increase in your own body's metabolism, plus the growth of your baby.

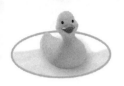

The Hebrew word for parents is *horim*, and it comes from the same root as *moreh*, teacher. The parent is, and remains, the first and most important teacher that the child will ever have.

—RABBI KASSEL ABELSON

_____

_____

_____

_____

_____

_____

_____

_____

_____

_____

_____

_____

_____

_____

_____

_____

_____

_____

_____

_____

_____

A HEALTHY
EXPECTATION
✦ ✦ ✦ ✦ ✦ ✦ ✦
The Fourth month:
Your precious baby
you are nurturing
will now be eight
inches long and
weighs six ounces.
The heartbeat is
strong and audible
with a stethoscope.
The baby may
occupy the time
now by sucking its
thumb. The skin is
forming into several
layers and is pink
and wrinkled. The
skeletal system is
thickening and
developing, and
some digestion
even begins this
month. The uterus
is greatly enlarging.

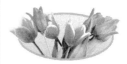

Listen to advice and accept instruction, and in the end you will be wise.

—PROVERBS 19:20

Lord, Help me to receive and take to heart the advice and instruction that lines up with Your Word. Give me the discernment to weigh the advice given to me and to make the right decisions for myself and for my baby.

A HEALTHY EXPECTATION
* * * * * * *

You have been created as the perfect host for your baby. You freely give—even without knowing you are—to whatever the need may be. Your formed placenta acts as a "screen," attempting to block the entry of toxic substances, but many unwanted substances can still get through to your baby. For this reason, your focus on what you eat and how you live allows you to serve as the healthy "gatekeeper" to your precious little one.

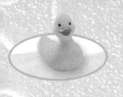

Being a successful parent requires that you speak two languages—yours and theirs.

—DAVID JEREMIAH

_____

_____

_____

_____

_____

_____

_____

_____

_____

_____

_____

_____

_____

_____

_____

_____

_____

_____

_____

_____

The food you eat
is the food that
makes your baby
healthy, happy,
and well nourished.
Such a blessed
baby starts life
with an advantage
that carries on
throughout a bright
future; every aspect
of your baby's life
will be affected by
the nutrition
received.

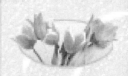

The mother's heart is the child's schoolroom.

—HENRY WARD BEECHER

_____

_____

_____

_____

_____

_____

_____

_____

_____

_____

_____

_____

_____

_____

_____

_____

_____

A HEALTHY EXPECTATION

＊　＊　＊　＊　＊　＊　＊

Life is a tremendous gift from God. We need to do everything we can to maximize this
precious gift. The best things we can give children are our time, our love, good habits,
and good memories.

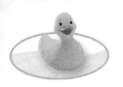

May the Lord make you increase, both you and your children. May you be blessed by the Lord, the Maker of heaven and earth.

—PSALM 115:14–15

_____

_____

_____

_____

_____

_____

_____

_____

_____

_____

_____

_____

_____

_____

_____

_____

_____

_____

_____

_____

_____

A HEALTHY
EXPECTATION
✦ ✦ ✦ ✦ ✦ ✦ ✦
Once you get your
day started with
breakfast, continue
to eat "minimeals"
often throughout
the day, about every
2 to 2½ hours.
Healthy and wise
snacking is like
throwing wood on a
fire throughout the
day to keep it
burning well. It will
result in more
energy, a healthy,
proper weight gain,
and will provide a
constant source of
nutrients in your
bloodstream to be
carried to the
placenta and your
baby.

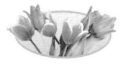

Who takes the child by the hand takes the mother by the heart.

—GERMAN PROVERB

A HEALTHY EXPECTATION
+ + + + + + +

The best way to assure your vitamin intake is to go for whole-grain carbohydrates
whenever possible, and choose meals full of a variety of brightly colored fruits and
vegetables. Vegetables and fruits are simple carbohydrates that provide a storehouse
of vitamins, minerals, and other substances for vitality living. They are also valuable
sources of fiber and fluids.

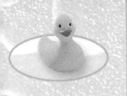

It's not the "IQ"
but the "I will" that
is important.

—ANONYMOUS

The good news is
this: If you are
eating the right
foods, at the right
times, in the right
balance—even with
a few splurges—
you will naturally
gain the right
amount of weight
in your pregnancy.
It's how your body
was created!

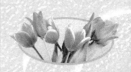

Pleasant words are a honeycomb, sweet to the soul and healing to the bones.

—PROVERBS 16:24

Father, may I speak pleasant words to my baby—and may my baby be formed
with words of life and love.

_____

_____

_____

_____

_____

_____

_____

_____

_____

_____

_____

_____

_____

_____

_____

_____

_____

_____

_____

_____

_____

_____

_____

_____

_____

_____

_____

_____

_____

_____

_____

_____

_____

_____

A HEALTHY EXPECTATION
✦ ✦ ✦ ✦ ✦ ✦ ✦

Close your eyes, take a deep breath, and put your hands over your womb. Send heart
messages of love and welcome to your baby growing inside. Do this several times a
day—rejoicing in the miracle of God.

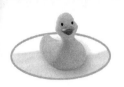

There is only one
truly beautiful baby
in the world, and
each mother has it.

—ANONYMOUS

_____
_____
_____
_____
_____
_____
_____
_____
_____
_____
_____
_____
_____
_____
_____
_____
_____
_____
_____

A HEALTHY EXPECTATION

✦ ✦ ✦ ✦ ✦ ✦ ✦

Leg cramps are
most common in
the second and
third trimesters,
and fatigue seems
to increase their
frequency. Give
your legs a break by
wearing support
hose during the
day, and take the
load off by resting
frequently
throughout the day
with your feet up.
Make sure your
calcium intake
stays high.

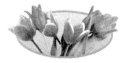

The illusions of childhood are necessary experiences: a child should not be denied a balloon because an adult knows that sooner or later it will burst.

—MARCELENE COX

A HEALTHY EXPECTATION
+ + + + + + +

The Fifth month: The angel is ten to twelve inches long and weighs fourteen to sixteen ounces. We finally got up to a pound. The baby is active now, and you may begin to feel the movement, known as "quickening," at about twenty weeks. A covering like peach fuzz appears over the entire body, and hair begins to grow. Internal organs are developing at an astonishing speed.

Every baby comes
with the message that
God is not yet
discouraged.

—ANONYMOUS

+ + + + + + +

Right up there with
what to name your
baby is the decision
of how best to feed
her. The decision to
breast or bottle-
feed your baby is
not one that can be
made under
pressure. This is
your baby's most
pleasurable time
with you; make it
enjoyable for both.
The most important
ingredient in
feeding your baby
is not what's given,
but that it's given
with love.

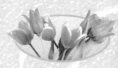

Father, I thank You for my unborn child. I treasure this child as a gift from You.
My child was created in Your image, perfectly healthy and complete.
You have known my child since conception and know the path my child will take in life.
I ask Your blessing, and stand in faith, believing Your plan for my child.

_____

_____

_____

_____

_____

_____

_____

_____

_____

_____

_____

_____

_____

_____

_____

_____

A HEALTHY EXPECTATION

♦ ♦ ♦ ♦ ♦ ♦ ♦

Pregnancy is a time of incredible demand on the body. For an overflow of energy, you
must give yourself the supply to meet these demands, and then some! Remember the
power of fueling with the eat-right prescription: right foods at the right time and in the
right balance—with lots of brightly colored fruits and veggies. And remember the
secret of *power snacking*—food through the day keeps fatigue at bay.

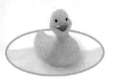

Insanity is hereditary; you get it from your children.

—SAM LEVENSON

_____

_____

_____

_____

_____

_____

_____

_____

_____

_____

_____

_____

_____

_____

_____

_____

_____

_____

_____

Should you ever
give in to cravings?
Honestly, in
pregnancy they are
almost a homicidal
drive—just try to
stop you! The goal
is to try to prevent
them by keeping
blood sugars
stable, nutrient and
fluid needs met—
and if they happen,
to make the best
of them by
choosing the
healthiest foods
you can.

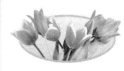

If your troubles aren't big enough to pray about,
then they certainly aren't big enough to fret about.

—ANONYMOUS

A HEALTHY EXPECTATION
＋ ＋ ＋ ＋ ＋ ＋ ＋

Fears can be the ugly side of pregnancy—the clouds that block the sunny days of anticipation. Talking about your concerns is a way to see them differently. Just getting them out of the whirlwind of your mind, out of the dark, can let you see them through the light and power of truth. Ask questions. Talk to friends. Journal. Pray.

Praise the Lord, O
my soul, and forget
not all his benefits.

—PSALM 103:2

_____

_____

_____

_____

_____

_____

_____

_____

_____

_____

_____

_____

_____

_____

_____

_____

_____

_____

_____

_____

_____

_____

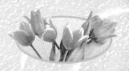

"I am like that" does not help anything. "I can be different" does.

—ANONYMOUS

_____

_____

_____

_____

_____

_____

_____

_____

_____

_____

_____

_____

_____

_____

_____

_____

A HEALTHY EXPECTATION
✦ ✦ ✦ ✦ ✦ ✦ ✦

Instead of looking at all you have to give up, set your eyes on what you are desiring to obtain: *I want a pregnancy filled with energy. I want a fit pregnancy. I want a body that works for me. I want to birth a baby who has been given nourishing food with love.*

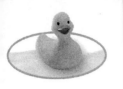

Ask your child
what he wants
for dinner only
if he's buying.

—FRAN LEBOWITZ

_____
_____
_____
_____
_____
_____
_____
_____
_____
_____
_____
_____
_____
_____
_____
_____
_____
_____
_____
_____

A HEALTHY
EXPECTATION
+ + + + + + +
Learn the ten best
and ten worst
foods. Increase your
intake of the best,
decrease or
eliminate your
intake of the worst,
and see how much
better you feel and
look! Get more of
the best foods into
your grocery cart
and your diet, and
you'll see a big
difference in your
energy, stamina,
hair, skin, nails, and
general well-being
right away. Looking
good and feeling
good come from
the inside.

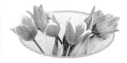

So God created man in his own image, in the image of God
he created him; male and female he created them.

Thank You, God, that this baby is being perfectly formed in Your image. May this baby share Your love, kindness, peace, forgiveness, hope, grace, and mercy with the world.

_____

_____

_____

_____

_____

_____

_____

_____

_____

_____

_____

_____

_____

_____

_____

_____

_____

_____

_____

_____

_____

_____

_____

_____

_____

_____

_____

_____

_____

_____

_____

_____

_____

_____

_____

_____

_____

_____

_____

_____

A HEALTHY EXPECTATION

✦ ✦ ✦ ✦ ✦ ✦ ✦

The Sixth month: Your baby now has fingerprints and footprints as the ridges on palms and soles of feet are fully formed. Sweet precious has now grown to a length of fourteen inches and weighs two pounds, which means you will gain slightly more weight during this month. You will be able to feel definite little friendly kicks as the baby makes you aware of its presence!

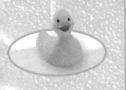

There are times
when parenthood
seems nothing but
feeding the mouth
that bites you.

—PETER DE VRIES

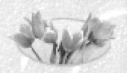

Wait for the Lord; be strong and take heart and wait for the Lord.

—PSALM 27:14

_____

_____

_____

_____

_____

_____

_____

_____

_____

_____

_____

_____

_____

_____

_____

_____

_____

_____

A HEALTHY EXPECTATION
+ + + + + + +

Constipation is very common in pregnancy, especially during the early weeks and again
toward the end. Be sure to get plenty of exercise and whole-grain carbohydrates,
specifically unprocessed wheat bran, fresh fruits, and leafy vegetables. Be sure to drink
adequate water (eight ounces before and after every meal and snack). You might try
filling a two-quart container with water each morning—be sure it's gone by bedtime.

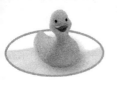

Worry doesn't empty tomorrow of its sorrows, it empties today of its strength.

—CORRIE TEN BOOM

_____

_____

_____

_____

_____

_____

_____

_____

_____

_____

_____

_____

_____

_____

_____

_____

_____

_____

_____

A HEALTHY EXPECTATION
♦ ♦ ♦ ♦ ♦ ♦ ♦
A cold or mild illness during your pregnancy may be uncomfortable, but it won't harm your baby. However, some of the medications you may normally take (like decongestants and antihistamines) could. So don't take anything—even extra vitamin C—without speaking to your doctor. You can get the most up-to-date list of the medications that are known to be safe—and the proper dosage for any symptoms you experience.

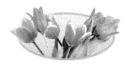

Nothing and no one can prevent God's plan from being fulfilled in your life [or that of your child] except your decision to give up on that plan.

—TOM NEWMAN

A HEALTHY EXPECTATION

✦ ✦ ✦ ✦ ✦ ✦ ✦

The Seventh month: The weight of your child has doubled since last month. Skin is red and wrinkled, but the fatty tissue begins to form underneath it and will fill it out to make it "soft as a baby's bottom." The baby is gaining about one-half pound a week now, and by the end of this month will weigh two-and-one-half to three-and-one-half pounds and will be about sixteen inches long. If born now, the baby could probably survive with special neonatal care, as the organ systems are well developed.

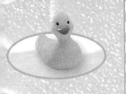

A mother should be like a quilt—keep the children warm but don't smother them.

—ANONYMOUS

If you are
experiencing
backaches, warm up
to pain relief—take
a long, warm bath,
morning and
evening, and try
applying a heating
pad wrapped in a
towel for up to
twenty minutes,
three or four times
a day. Most of all,
relax. Many back
problems are
aggravated by
stress and tension.

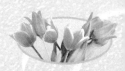

A lasting work requires extensive preparation.

—DOUGLAS RUMFORD

_____

_____

_____

_____

_____

_____

_____

_____

_____

_____

_____

_____

_____

_____

_____

_____

_____

_____

A HEALTHY EXPECTATION
+ + + + + + +

Proverbs tells us that "[S]he who refreshes others will [herself] be refreshed" (Prov. 11:25, NIV). This cannot be truer than when you are providing the very best for your baby. You sow—and both the baby and you reap!

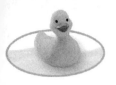

So do not fear, for I am with you; do not be dismayed, for I am your God. I will strengthen you and help you; I will uphold you with my righteous right hand.

—ISAIAH 41:10

Lord, help me to know that I am not alone in labor—that I need not fear being unable to "get through." I receive Your promise that You will strengthen and help me.

_____

_____

_____

_____

_____

_____

_____

_____

_____

_____

_____

_____

_____

_____

_____

_____

You are
experiencing one of
the biggest
transition periods
of your life—and
many emotions,
both positive and
negative, will rise to
the surface.
Processing these
emotions is vital to
your emotional—
and physical—well-
being.

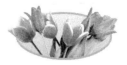

If I had a single flower for everytime I think about you (my precious baby), I could walk forever in my garden.

—CLAUDIA GRANDI

A HEALTHY EXPECTATION
+ + + + + + +

Keeping active while you are pregnant can be as beneficial to you psychologically as it is physically. Most woman find that exercise reduces the aches and pains associated with pregnancy and boosts their energy levels and self-esteem. You will probably get back into shape faster and more easily after delivery if you've kept your body in good condition during your pregnancy.

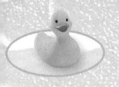

Come unto me, all that labour and are heavy laden, and I will give you rest.

—MATTHEW 11:28, KJV

Lord, Help me to remember that it isn't the load that weighs me down, but the way I carry it. . . .

_____

_____

_____

_____

_____

_____

_____

_____

_____

_____

_____

_____

_____

_____

_____

_____

_____

_____

_____

_____

_____

A HEALTHY EXPECTATION

✦ ✦ ✦ ✦ ✦ ✦

Workouts don't have to be elaborate, just regular. In fact, a gentle walking program and some basic stretching can be your first step toward a lifetime of fitness. It's something we all know how to do, you can do it anywhere, and the only equipment you need is a comfortable pair of shoes.

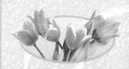

Worry is like sitting in a rocking chair.
It gives you something to do, but it doesn't get you anywhere.

—ANONYMOUS

_____
_____
_____
_____
_____
_____
_____
_____
_____
_____
_____
_____
_____
_____
_____
_____
_____
_____
_____
_____

A HEALTHY EXPECTATION
+ + + + + + +

Begin each exercise session with five to ten minutes of low-intensity exercise such as
walking. Complete your warmup or cool down by stretching calves, chest, lower back,
and hamstrings. Hold each stretch for twenty seconds without bouncing. For cool
downs, increase the stretch time to thirty seconds.

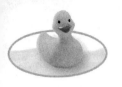

It's tough to fly with the eagles in the morning when you stay up all night with the owls.

—ANONYMOUS

_____

_____

_____

_____

_____

_____

_____

_____

_____

_____

_____

_____

_____

_____

_____

_____

_____

_____

_____

A HEALTHY EXPECTATION

✦ ✦ ✦ ✦ ✦ ✦ ✦

The power of the afternoon nap cannot be overstated. Just twenty minutes of sleep can do miracles for regenerating the body. If you can't sleep, just lie down (remember, on the left side!) with a good book. If you are at an office, use your break times as a time to sit quietly with your feet up on a desk or resting in the ladies lounge. If you already have children, discipline yourself to nap when they nap— and to ignore the laundry.

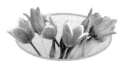

It is not now troubled the sea that determines the course of your life; it is who the Pilot is.

—ANONYMOUS

A HEALTHY EXPECTATION

✦ ✦ ✦ ✦ ✦ ✦ ✦

Heartburn can be controlled by eating in an evenly distributed way throughout the day, helping to keep gastric acids neutralized. Do not resort to antacids! Remember—eat to prevent heartburn rather than trying to treat it once it's started.

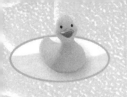

I lift up my eyes to the hills—where does my help come from? My help comes from the Lord, the Maker of heaven and earth.

—PSALM 121:1

_____

_____

_____

_____

_____

_____

_____

_____

_____

_____

_____

_____

_____

_____

_____

_____

_____

_____

_____

_____

_____

A HEALTHY EXPECTATION

◆ ◆ ◆ ◆ ◆ ◆ ◆

Treat herbal remedies as you would any drug during pregnancy. Simply do not take them unless directed to do so by your doctor. Don't even drink herbal teas. If you have symptoms that need treatment, seek the advice of your practitioner—do not treat yourself—and don't listen to your Aunt Susie!

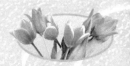

When was the last time that your children saw you on your knees with an open Bible seeking direction from God? That is an unmistakable lesson to a child.

—CHARLES STANLEY

_____

_____

_____

_____

_____

_____

_____

_____

_____

_____

_____

_____

_____

_____

_____

_____

_____

_____

_____

A HEALTHY EXPECTATION
+ + + + + + +

The Eighth month: As more fat is deposited under the skin, the baby reaches about
five pounds in weight and eighteen inches in length. Lungs develop strength.
Soon you will hear that wailing you've been waiting for. The brain continues its
rapid development, with the cells multiplying at a rapid rate.

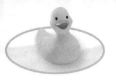

Put off thy cares
with thy clothes;
so shall thy rest
strengthen thy labor,
and so thy labor
sweeten thy rest.

—FRANCIS QUARLES

If you find yourself
waking up during
the night or
sleeping restlessly,
be sure that you
have a bedtime
snack that will keep
your blood sugar
levels more even as
you sleep. It will
keep you sleeping
more deeply, and
will prevent a
lighter state of
sleep that acutely
makes you aware of
baby aerobics, full
bladders, and
general discomfort.

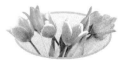

May the Lord bless and protect you; may the Lord's face radiate with joy because of you;

may he be gracious to you, show his favor, and give you his peace.

—NUMBERS 6:24–26, TLB

A HEALTHY EXPECTATION

* * * * * * *

If you have difficulty going to sleep at night, be sure to get adequate exercise during the day; an evening walk followed by a warm shower does wonders! Also, be sure that you position yourself with lots of pillows for maximum comfort. Many women find that sleeping on their side with a pillow between their knees is a very comfortable position.

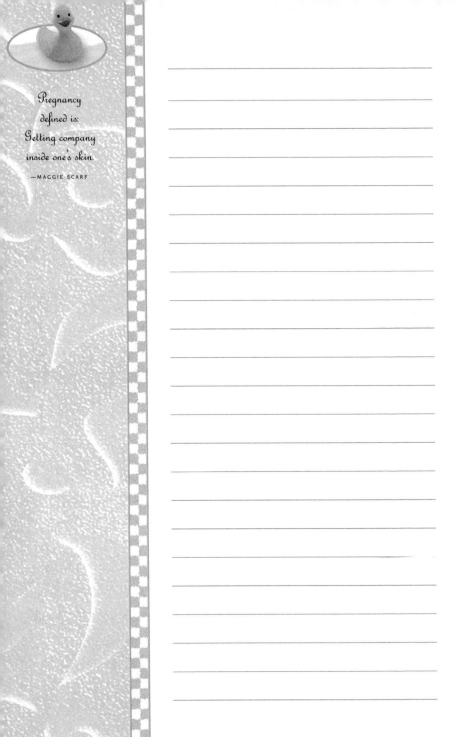

Pregnancy
defined is:
Getting company
inside one's skin.

—MAGGIE SCARF

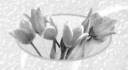

"Everything is permissible for me"—but not everything is beneficial. "Everything is permissible for me"—but I will not be mastered by anything.

A HEALTHY EXPECTATION
• • • • • • •

Everyone requires some sodium and, although your need for it during pregnancy
actually increases, there's more than enough sodium naturally present in foods to
supply this requirement. Sodium should not be severely restricted during pregnancy,
but if you use salt to an extreme, it would be wise to cut back on its overuse. Become
aware of where you may be using salt in excess.

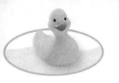

You have to love
your children
unselfishly.
That's hard, but
it's the only way.

—BARBARA BUSH

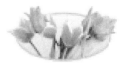

Heavenly Father, You are my refuge; I trust You during this time of waiting.
I am thankful that You have put angels at watch over me and my unborn child.
I cast all care and burden for this pregnancy and birth over onto You.
Your grace is sufficient for me. You strengthen my weaknesses. Amen

A HEALTHY EXPECTATION
✦ ✦ ✦ ✦ ✦ ✦ ✦
Take time for soul care. Whether your trip is for a day, a weekend, or a week,
look for an opportunity to get away from the normal distractions of life—leave some
time to reflect on the many changes taking place within, and make some significant
spiritual connections.

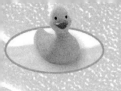

The real message in dealing with a five-year-old is that in no time at all, you will begin to sound like a five-year-old.

—JEAN KERR

_____

_____

_____

_____

_____

_____

_____

_____

_____

_____

_____

_____

_____

_____

_____

_____

_____

_____

A HEALTHY EXPECTATION
♦ ♦ ♦ ♦ ♦ ♦ ♦
Varicose veins can be prevented or their symptoms minimized by wearing support pantyhose, elevating your legs when you are sitting, avoiding prolonged standing, avoiding excessive weight gain, and exercising (in moderation) thirty minutes a day. Gentle aerobic exercises like walking, swimming, or exercise-biking will divert blood from the venous system back towards the heart.

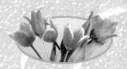

I rise before dawn and cry for help; I have put my hope in your word.

—PSALM 119:147

_____

_____

_____

_____

_____

_____

_____

_____

_____

_____

_____

_____

_____

_____

_____

_____

_____

_____

A HEALTHY EXPECTATION

✦ ✦ ✦ ✦ ✦ ✦ ✦

If you are experiencing any symptoms that necessitate a call to your doctor,
mention everything you're feeling—even if it seems unrelated. Describe how
long and how frequently the symptoms have occurred, if anything has
relieved the symptoms, and how severe they are.

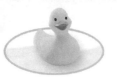

"I know the plans
I have for you,"
declares the Lord,
"plans to prosper
and not to harm you,
plans to give you
hope and a future."

—JEREMIAH 29:11

✦ ✦ ✦ ✦ ✦ ✦ ✦

The Ninth month:
By delivery time
your baby will
weigh an average of
seven pounds and
measure twenty to
twenty-one-inches
long. Your baby's
biggest weight gain
will occur during
this last month. It
will store iron, fat-
soluble vitamins,
and minerals as
reserves after birth
and is also building
up immunities.
That little darling is
now ready and
waiting to join its
family.

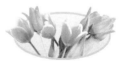

But our families will continue; generation after generation
will be preserved by your protection.

—PSALM 102:28, TLB

Lord, I pray not only for the baby growing within me right now, but I pray for all my descendants that they'll love and serve You. Teach me how to raise my baby with a thirst for righteousness that will be passed down from generation to generation.

A HEALTHY EXPECTATION
✦ ✦ ✦ ✦ ✦ ✦ ✦

Your body took nine months to expand, and it will take three to nine months to shed all your weight and get back into your normal-best form. Whether you breastfeed or bottle-feed, the most important things you can do after giving birth are to heal, stay as healthy and energized as you can, and take the best possible care of that sweet baby.

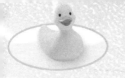

About Your New Baby

Baby's full name _____

We chose this name for our baby because _____

_____

_____

Date of birth _____

Time of birth _____

Weight at birth _____

Length at birth _____

Color and amount of hair _____

Any distinguishing marks? _____

Any unique birth experiences? _____

Was the baby born on the due date? _____

Days early _____ Days late _____

What did you do the first time you held your baby?

_____

_____

_____

Describe your baby's first feeding experience.

_____

_____

_____

Other books by Pamela Smith:

Healthy Expectations

The Good Life—A Healthy Cookbook

Eat Well—Live Well

Food For Life

Come Cook With Me

Alive and Well in the Fast Lane

For more information about Pamela Smith's books, tapes, speaking, and seminar/workshops please write or call:

PAMELA M. SMITH, R.D.
P.O. Box 541009
Orlando, FL 32854
800.896.4010 (orders)
407.855.8630 (information)

or

CREATION HOUSE
600 Rinehart Road
Lake Mary, FL 32746
800.599.5750
(Fax) 800.283.4561